He cured his Cancer!!!!!

Lesley my friend said, and she continued:

It has been almost 6 years now...No surgery and no chemo and no radiation, just good organic food, and sunshine, some saunas....Some vitamins and supplements!

Lesley said -He looks vibrant and healthier than anyone I know!

Lesley continued:

Such an ordeal it was, my life changed and James's life changed so much! All the goal setting and all the whatever and control over the way of life went out the

window! I had thought I would continue working & living in the Bay Area where I had such a nice life or at least I thought I did and I thought I was in control of my life!

Everything changed once we got the news!!!! With a huge news like CANCER, especially when your loved one has been diagnosed with it!

First, you get all confused, then sad and angry and...Then you take steps intended to get things done right!!! What is right? Who knows? Lots of research and whatever makes sense, the first thing is to not believe a word anyone says! No one really knows unless they have gone through it and succeeded, otherwise it is just another opinion coming from maybe EGO!

We are so lucky to have access to the information that is out there at our fingertips, why believe and react to people who just like to talk?

While doctors know so much, they get the same diseases and they die of the samethings!!! Just look at them, many are overweight and sick themselves and they tell us what to eat and what to do...They follow the books and they follow the systems set up for them and they follow the money and EGO!!!

I started asking myself intending to ask GOD, what should I do and where do I start from?
I kept asking, my fear was not allowing the information to come to me, or at least I was getting information in small pieces...

Once the diagnosis come, they (doctors) keep rushing you, scaring you and they keep on ....Never forget the patient holds the key, sometimes we have to make the hardest decision, not the easiest!
Never forget GOD and Love, in the absence of love (God) fear will take over. Making decisions with fear is deadly!!!!

James graduated from UCLA engineering Dept with honor and later took the test & signed up to go to another top University in the area to become a dentist,
with a great GPA and a great DAT score, I was very hopeful about his future.
I remember his graduation day at UCLA, I can easily say it was one of the best days of my life. James was happy himself too.
His accomplishment with honor, that was something fantastic!

How many people go to school and do not graduate, and so many do not even go.

I went back and forth to Los Angeles a few times a year while he was going to UCLA and I did the same thing again while he was going to USC.

For Holidays James would come home and sometimes in the summer too. I visited him often, on his birtdays and many other occasions.

I remember when he was attending UCLA he was happy
and he was taking care of himself well.

It was not the same with this other school, I found him stressed out often. At times he was not even taking time to talk to me. When I went for a visit he wanted me to leave and go home fast.

After a year James dropped out of USC, this was after incurring about $100K of student loan. He had issues with the crazy way the school staff had handled him.

Lesley said, When my son James told me the way he was treated, I said to him- I wish you would have dropped out in 2 months, not in 12 months! He said- I had to make sure I am doing the right thing and giving it my best shut!!!! I thought such courage! I said to him- You are an engineer any way & no one can take that away from you! I saw a shadow of confirmation looks on his face! He said I worked so hard all of my life, did all the right things and now this!!!

He moved to Vegas to have a fun life! He was also working as a tutor online and making a living that way.

I went to Vegas a few times visiting him, he was not happy. James had gained weight, I can easily say he was over weight.
I am not sure what was going on with him.

About a year and a half later he came home for a visit, to Los Gatos, where I lived. After a while he wanted to get some kind of work, tried a few things and chose not to go for them and still was earning a living as a tutor.

Lesley had tears in her eyes and continued:

It was the first week of September, one day he said-mom what do you think this is? He was showing me something on his neck, a walnut-size growth, I was terrified and could not believe it, he was too!

He went for a checkup and after a few days, the doctor called him and said he got the result and he wants to see him on Friday. We were both concerned why is he not telling and wants to see him? That must be???

It was that Friday afternoon I got out of work and I was supposed to meet a friend that I had not seen in decades, I met my friend and a few minutes later James called, he could hardly talk. He was devastated and said the doctor said it is Cancer... I was devastated ...I said I will be home right away, Please go home and I will see you in 30 minutes. My friend understood that I was in trouble & I have to go...I left to go home to see my son!

When I got home, he was not there...Not there for an hour or two...And my mind went crazy, I kept bringing my thoughts to something reasonable and even I was praying and asking God to help him and help me...

After an hour or two he showed up, we both had tears in our eyes and I hugged him and told him I loved him and asked him where he was ...He said he had just sat in his car and could not even drive and he had to put

himself together ...

We were both crushed! I knew I had to be strong and be good support, I said to him- Anytime we get a cut anywhere, like, I was showing my hand, even if we do not do anything it will get healed by itself, we must have something in our body to do that, I saw a bit of hope on his face.

I called my friend Elize, Doc Elize, she does alternative medicine work, she came by the house and spent a few hours with James, then we went to her house and we bought a lot of supplements and organic helping things from her.

I said to my son whatever decision you make I am with you 100%! He looked at me. I asked him to go for a 2nd opinion, he said ok and I went with him. We went to a doctor in San Francisco, he confirmed that was the

Thyroid Cancer.

This doctor was suggested by a friend of mine who was misdiagnosed to have cancer by another doctor 10 years ago and this doctor had told him he did not have cancer and the friend was Ok...That is why we

chose him. Hoping he will say the same to James.
This doctor confirmed it was cancer, after that
confirmation he sent us to the specialist at UCSF, we
went there.
 The waiting room was so bad, bad energy, sadness
was on most faces...
They had Chocolate kisses and other sweet things
on different tables...Did I wonder why? Isn't sugar
the worst thing for cancer? I noticed some people
reaching out for the sweets... Finally, James was
called & I ask to go in with him too and he said OK...
The way the specialist, the doctor was talking was
almost sounding as if he was excited!!!!
He was explaining how he will cut & then treat with
chemo...He went on & on and he continued that in
a year or two it may come back, then he will cut
more & use radiation for...& more Chemo...I was getting sick to my stomach and I kept reminding myself I have to be strong so James can lean on me!
I just could not believe James's strength listening to
this specialist! After a while James stood up from his
seat and said to the doctor- I am going to take my
time and do my own research and then decide if I
need you I will come back and see you.
The doctor got all out of shape, no, no, you have to
do this right away, James said no I am not going to
do this now, I think by January I will make my decision, (about 3 months). Although I was scared I
thought wow how courageous my son is...The doc-

tor kept saying how fast this will grow & many scary things and James said I will see you if I need you. The doctor said if you don't like me to do the surgery I will recommend another
specialist, another doctor, a great referral, he mentioned a name and said he can also do a fine job...You have to do this as soon as possible.
I thought I have to interfere, it was becoming like an
argument & maybe even loud, I said - Doctor do you really think within 3 months this will be life threatening? He said yes & no ...
James still said - Some times in January I will make my decision and we got out of there...

It felt like my heart was bleeding I was crushed! I kept thinking, I am not James and I feel so awful, what about him?
I was scared and I was relieved because his decision gave me some hope too...Knowing the numbers to be so bad when Patients go for Chemo & Surgery! Not only that, how sick they get with surgery ....And the
longterm effect and life-changing conditions, wow removing thyroid gland?
How crazy that is?

When we got home, I said- I am 100% with whatever you decide and I am not able to say what is a better way. It is about your life, and I do not know at all...It is your decision. I continued - Know that I am with you 100%.

One of James's student's dad had said to him a while back a few things about organic foods VS nonorganic foods...How pesticide causes cancer and many other
diseases...James explained that to me and we went totally organic and James decided no animal products at all anymore! We would go shopping at the health food stores.
 I was thinking I will do whatever it takes to give him hope & support. Once shopping at the WF he saw the cashier spraying the surface of the area where we were emptying the cart to, so he put his veggies & fruits on top of the bags and when the cashier almost put the broccoli on the contaminated surface, James took the broccoli away from him. He said to the cashier, these are organic foods and your cleaning spray are chemical, the cashier said yes, that is how we clean the area, what do you suggest to do? James said please just use vinegar & water. The cashier was a nice guy said wow that is good, I think that should work... I will also tell my manager that is what we should do here.
I was so impressed with my son!

For a few weeks, he stopped working, mainly because he could not think straight then he started again, I was happy for him deciding to go back to work. That gave me more hope.

James would boil organic potatoes and eat vegetables and fruits only. He would drink filtered water only, we put reverse osmoses by our kitchen sink.

Within 2 months he lost the extra 45 pounds and the tumor looked like it was shrinking too.
 James looked so good, he would go to saunas a few times a week to get the toxins out of his body and he was working out every day as well. We would go on long hikes a few times a week.
James bought a small and portable Sauna to use at home too, he knew the importance of getting heavy metal and toxins out his body by using the sauna often.

It was around the Holidays ... James did not want to see any relatives or anybody. He said they would say things to interfere with his decision, so we went to the beach to Shell Beach areas...
We took Highway one towards South, I had not driven the coastlines for many years. I had forgotten how it can becomes so hard especially at night.
Once the driver behind me had his high beams on and I was going blind and I changed the lane and

went to the right, somthing told me to stop com-
pletely and
immediatly, and I did even though I was thinking a
car may hit me from the back! It was a miracle that
I stopped, otherwise the car and us in it would have
fallen off the cliff! I was horified!! Almost paral-
ized with fear.
James guided me to get out of that area and get back
to the road and said not to pay attention to crazy
drivers.

I turned the mirror to stop seeing the blinding
lights! I kept driving. My SUV had too much EMF
(Elctro
Magnatic Field) radition in the front seat area, and
James would sit in the back seat and would not
drive my car. Finally we got to one of those coastal
towns, we had to find a place to stay for the night
and this was the busy time of the year, we got lucky
and found a room in a small hotel by the beach.

We were both so preoccupied by the health issues
we had not made any plans. We had not even made a
reservation. We had no plan to where to go and
what to do ...Just driving away to see where we end
up!

It seemed we were being guided by our higher
power, the few days by the beach went by very well.

We spent time walking on the beach, sitting in the sun when sun
became available or just sat by the ocean under the clouds.

Walking by the ocean, on the sand barefoot was so good for James, he said he was grounding his body, earthing, and getting rid of electricity and other toxins that way, and neutralizing his body and his cells.

Although I am not sophisticated enough with chimstry and physics these were making sense to me somewhat.

A few days later we were back at home. James was thinking Los Gatos is too congested we need to live somewhere less crowded and more peaceful and with more space. So we were both thinking where we should go and how we can manage doing the things we might need to do.

I was still working every work day...I did not know what to do, we had our ups and downs ...A huge generation gap!!! Mom & Son! I kept looking at the light at the end of the tunnel and seeing him well!!!

I would not have tears in my eyes when I was around him. My co worker's daughter had the same thing a few months before this, and she had surgery &

Chemo...

I was reading & doing research as well as James!
I remember reading about a few people with the same diagnosis, after two or three years they had all died except the one who had changed her lifestyle and had changed her diet & added yoga and meditation, even though this young lady had done chemo & surgery she was surviving. The survivor had decided to go
alternative after the chemo treatment. That was the only survivor in that article.

Then I found out about Suzzane S, an actress, in fact, she had written a book about how she almost died after surgery and Chemo. She changed her way of life, food and everything that could get absorbed to her body were all organic now. That is how she beat her cancer and got her life back!

Right before Christmas James said we should move to Northern CA. somewhere less congested, I said Ok, I tried to transfer my work to Santa Rosa, very quickly I was transferred, but I took a week off, James found us a place in San Rafael area. My boss wanted me to work at San Rafel banking Center. I was one of the top
producers in the San Jose area, this way I could be helping that center with loans in that area. I was

a mortgage loan officer. Santa Rosa office was the main office and was not too far.

We moved to that place, it was a rental for 45 days. It was only to see what to do. James continued with healthy eating, vegan, organic and sunbathing, sauna, and walking every day for a few miles while I was

working.

One of the girls at work told me about her friend's husband a 28 year man with two small children was also diagnosed with cancer a few months ago. The young man was being pressured by everyone including the lady who was telling me about him to go through the surgery and Chemo therapy like most people do. She was saying he was taking care of it the natural way by organic food. She said he was losing weight, she was talking about him as if he is doing it wrong. I have not found out what happened to him at all!

Lesley my friend was tearful most of the time while she was talking. I was so interested to know more. She continued: My head was not working, my business was not getting anywhere. I decided to tell my story to a total stranger that I was working with and asked her to tell me what to do since my head was not telling me. She saw my tears and she knew I was really in trouble ....First she said she does not know what to say... I asked again- What would you do if you were me? My head is not working I am full of fear...

She thought for a while, then she said to take a family leave, she said with the family leave of absence you can get paid 75% of your income while taking care of

your loved one. She suggested to do it right away and not waste anytime!

This was almost the end of Feb. 2014, I took a day to decided & I did it.

I shocked James and I shocked my boss! I decided to take a family leave of absence, I had never done anything like this before!

Amazingly God works in mysterious ways. I was at the social security age, by about 4 months away from 66 and I had some savings. I thought if anything bad

happens to James I will never forgive myself that I could be there for him full time and I did not do it...So I should do this. Even if I spend all of my life savings it will be worth to help my son, I can always get a job of some kind once he gets well again. His life is the most

important and I have to treat it that way...

When I put the effort in anything it always works out the best, I have to do it!

So I did that. I took a leave of abscence. This was end

of February 2014.

None of the rental places we had looked at worked out. Some of them were near farms and greenaries and we could smell the pesticides and we were trying to get away from the poisons. The ones in the middle of the towns had other issues, as if God had other plans for us.
Our 45 days rental time was up, and we had no place to rent in that area.
We had to leave the rental place in Marine County.
We had found out Marin County had one of the highest cancer rates in the nation because of something they had dumped in the ocean of that area after the war. I really had just heard that and did not really know for sure.

We went to my friend's house in Pleasanton to stay a few weeks to give ourselves time to think about and see where we should go...

January had come and gone, it seemed James knew what he was doing.
In Pleasanton very quickly we found out about the Lawrence Livermore Lab. It is close to pleasanton. We learned stories about radiation and contamination of certain areas that some workers of that research Lab had dumped radioactive materials on those certain areas near by.

Amazingly all of these very expensive areas had their own issues and most people were not aware of them and / or not paying attention.

After some research, I found out that almost everywhere in the US, most cities and towns are about 10 to 50 miles away from a nuclear facility, power plant or a nuclear dump site! Although I did not check every town or city it seemed that way to me.

We found out the only place far enough would be Palm Springs which is 110 miles away from the closest one in San Onofre. We also read about San Onofre's leakage problem.
Instead of staying in Pleasanton for a month, within a week we drove to Palm Springs area. We stayed in short term rentals.

It was a different lifestyle, we were about 20-25 miles away from Palm Springs in a country setting, about 2800 feet elevation, mountains everywhere, beautiful views!! We could see the beautiful sky full of stars at night ...Amazing settings, wild rabbits everywhere, birds were singing ...There was no greenery and therefore no pesticides!!!! High desert area. Lots of sunshine.

I had a very panicky feeling for a while, I had always worked and now, no work! It was a different feeling and it took me a while to get used to it and slow down a bit.

In Palm Springs area, we met some nice and some strange people. Very quickly we learned to guard our emotions, there were people who said so many stories about their knowledge and expertise, we found out it was only ego.

we met a nice young doctor and his girl friend who lived next door to us, the young doctor about 30 years old, was recovering from a major stomach surgery. He said he only has 1/3 of his stomach left and most his
digestive system, intestines were cutoff, he was very sick.

I do not think he gave himeself any chance to learn about his body, I saw him falling a few times. He was very weak. Oonce I offered him some natural, organic cherry juice, he loved it. He told me some-how that juice helped him a lot, he wanted to know where I bought it from. I gave him the small heath food place information. He went there and came back with many things, he said he did not know about the natural foods that he can eat instead of the junk he has been eating.
He said he loves the cherry juice more than the regular soft drinks!

A few days later they left the vacation rental and went home.

We also left the vacation rental and rented a house, a

small house in Joshua Tree and moved there. I do not know what happened to that young doctor, I hope

he survived.

There were so many great hiking places there in Joshua Tree, we were hiking everyday.

The National Park itself is a great place to go hiking and we did go there a lot too.

After a few weeks, James got a Cannabis Medical License for his personal medical use. It was very hard for him but it looked like it was helping at times it looked like it was shrinking the tumor, but not really.

James was sunbathing every day, falling sleep everywhere because of the Cannabis.

We had changed everything our soaps, shampoos, and cleaning stuff. Everything we were using was organic and had no smell. It was a new way of living!

After 2 months of using Cannabis, when James went to get his new supply, he was shocked, with the first try he knew it was not the same thing, he took it back and did not want to continue with cannabis at all anymore.

January had come and gone a few months ago, I was happy to know James had already made his decision and he was not going back to the doctors again.

Somehow I knew he was healed, James looked very healthy and very good, great sense of humor and happy. I had heard you clean your liver your life will change, I think that was happening to James. We were juicing every day and eating the good stuff.

I was going back & forth to the Bay area to rent out my house in Los Gatos, so my mortgage would be taken care of. Happily I was able to do that.

I sold the condo I owned in West LA that gave me some money, I Put a huge down payment on a house with 1.5 acre of land and I bought the house with the seller
financing the loan.
Now about almost a year later after the diagnosis, I felt James had made a great decision not getting involved with the medical ways...My son looking great, healthy, but that tumor was still there, not getting bigger but was there!

I had found out I was not going to get paid at all,

my family leave was not approvable as hard as I had tried.

Since James was not using a regular medical system the insurance company and my work were not approving my family leave of absence!

This was shocking to me, Even though the diagnosis and the lab tests were all there Just because he was not going to a doctor for help & treatment they had turned down my family leave, and I was not getting paid other than my monthly Social Security payments.

After that, my boss had asked me to resign and I did. Then I tried to get unemloyment benefits but that one was also turned down.

My son was healthy again! That was much more important than getting paid, but how sad is the system!!! I could not get paid for something everyone gets paid when they take care of a family member,

because James was not being treated by the doctors?!!!!!

I thought It is Ok...I have my son, he is getting better, he is saving his life I do not need that money ...I will do whatever I have to do!

We were juicing, he was eating the potatoes, vegetables & fruits, and sun bathing ...Wow what a great way to heal!

After we moved to the house in September, within a month James decided to go to South America. He said the southern hemisphere has cleaner air because there is the Amazon Jungle.   James said the population is about 75% less there and the filter is about 80% more there, so cleaner air & everything! He had bought all kinds of gadgets for EMF (Electro Magnetic Field) of all kinds, and filtration. He was not going to fly to So. America because the higher atmosphere has so much radiation, so he was looking at the alternative way of travel.

I decided to go with him. He was happy about that and he suggested to go on a cruise and we did and we went to Ecuador. Although the cruise was nice, he was

targeted by the crew because he had many electronic gadgets.

 It was so horrifying to deal with them. There, we were on the ship and we had to deal with this?! After they checked everything, they left us alone!

We were both worried about the crazy things that have happened on the cruise lines. We had heard stories ...So we decided we will go everywhere together neither one of us was going anywhere alone while we were on the ship.

 It was an 11 days cruise finally we got to Manta, our destination!

Manta was shockingly a poor looking port!
From Manta we took a shuttle to a coastal city called Guayaquil, it was many hours on the shuttle until we got there. The 3rd world was so obvious to us in that long drive. We saw the things we had only seen in the movies before. Very poor, in many ways. The people
living in basic ways. Very old people were carrying heavy things and trying to sell things. The bathrooms had no toilet papers. I learned quicky to buy my own toilet paper and take some with me.

We did not speak Spanish but we had a small translator gadget with us, that was somewhat helpful. Some people spoke broken English and that was helpful.

Guayaquil was so humid and hot, it was a big city with a lot of traffic. We met a taxi driver who spoke good
English and he gave us some good information. We got a nice hotel to stay the night and a good restaurant to eat at and a great market for James to buy his produce.

We took a bus to go to Cuenca, another big city. Many people from all over the world go there. Many Americans live there too.   The bus ride was some

kind of adventurous, a big bus driving on top of the
mountains, on very narrow roads! Wonderful
sceneries, green, huge mountains, many water-
falls....Wow how beautiful these places were! At
times we wondered, if we were going to get to
Cuenca in one piece, and safe, it was scary...

Cuenca itself was not bad, it was another develop-
ing city. We got a place to stay for the night and
walked down the street to get produce and may be
some food. Some of these restaurants would prepare potatoes for James too.
At the restaurant the owner came and sat with us,
he told us about a cute town called Vilcabamba he
said there are many young people there. Many
Americans live there. He said it is about 4 or 5 hours
away. He suggested to take the shuttle and go there
to see.

He spoke English well. He described the town to us,
we decided to go there. We went there the next day,
it took us a half a day. We took a shuttle to Loja and
then a taxi to Vilcabmba.
We stayed in a hosteria for that day and night, it was
OK.

The next morning we decided to walk around and
check things out. We kept walikng up the mountain
road. Right by the river, it was so refreshing. After

walking for about 2 miles, we saw a "for rent" sign.

We asked to see the house for rent. It was a cute little house in the back of a property, A large property with two houses on it. The property was by the river, it was a very nice setting.
The owner lived on the same property. The owners were a family with 3 children and few dogs and chickens and roosters.

They lived in the big house in front and the back house was the small house and seemed very safe. James rented it right away, the price was unbeliveably good.
Very nice peope , they had many cages for many animals...
Vilcabamba was a cute little town with many modern buildings, many people spoke English.
Many restaurants & shopps. People from all over the world were living there. Many American, German, and many from other countries too.
Once James was setteled in, I left and came back to California.
He liked the town Vilcabamba so he asked me to prepare his paperwork for residency & send them to him. It took a while and I did the work. He had already started some of the work before we went to Ecuador so I was able to do it.

I did not know what to do in So. California by my-self.

James and I were both poker players, we played on-line.

We were both very good at it, we were both making a few hundred dollars a month playing poker. I could check his poker table online and it was very comforting to know that we had that game to play & I could watch him play online from California to Vilcabamba.

I decided to go and live near my son in Vilcabamba.

To do this I had to make my life simpler. That meant I had to sell my house in Los Gatos and pay off the mortgage of my house in So. California.

I listed my house with an agent in Los Gatos, things did not work out.

I got an offer but it was not good and my agent made a few big mistakes.

I took the listing back and gave the listing to my sister to sell it for me. She is a broker, I was hoping this will give me less headache and more peace of mind.

My sister was not doing good financially at that time and this would help her too.

Long story short I almost lost everything, my sister was very reckless with my tenant and my property.

I had to pay the mortgage payments from my savings since she got rid of the rent paying tenant of mine!
Almost lost everything.   The very first offer I got from her I sold the house, to just end the problems.
I paid off my mortgage, and simplified my life. Even though I lost good amount of money.

 I prepared my papers ready for residency in Ecuador and, then I flew back about March of 2015 to Quito and then went to Vilcabamba Ecuador.

James was doing great, looking healthy and well and fit! Although he was not depressed he was very cautious and thoughtful. At times he would say he can not figure out why this tumor is not going away...
He was using baking soda, lemon and vinegar regularly and sunshine every day...He was working online and making some money.
I was enjoying myself there too...The weather was so nice...No chemtrails. The air was clean and crisp.

There was a Farmers Marker on Saturdays, all organic
produce and many organic shops for the rest of the week.
I was taking Spanish lessons, and meeting new people.   I was walking to James's house up the

mountain everyday. I lived in down town area so it would take me awhile to walk to James's place up on the mountain.

One day James walked over to my house with a cute little poppy. I was so happy for him, now the little poppy will ease his mind and that will be great.
The dog was adorable, he named her Mia. He took her everywhere with him. She turned out to be a beautiful dog, German Shepherd and Colli mix.

I was learning about So. America and healthier way of living.
About September 2015 James was telling me he was getting very board and wanting to move back to California.

We had to go to Peru to get to the Ship, and take that cruise again. It was December of 2015. We had to make the dog, Mia, a service dog to be able to take her with us on the cruise.
After so many buses, and so many hotels in so many days, finally we got to Lima Peru...Everything worked out good even though it was not easy at all!
We met a very nice man who helpped us a lot and he spoke English very well.
It is amazing how many great people show up to help!
It took us over a week to travel the coastal areas to

get to Lima Peru. Once we got to the ship it got easier. The cruise was for 18 days ....We had many nice stops along the way...We somehow managed the trip well.

Once we got back to California, it took us a few days to settle again. It was Christmas and New Year time.

I noticed James was healthier than ever before, looking great, I thought I should leave him alone and let him find himself again after the huge ordeal!

I left James and his dog Mia & went back to Ecuador...I came back and forth often and noticed his emotional improvements.

In March of 2017 When I came back I found him in love & happier than ever before...

Love is the key to all the great things in life...

Unfortunately it did not last, they broke up...

His health was excellent but that tumor was still there, maybe a bit smaller. Even though the relationship did not last that feeling opened many doors for James. He seemed to be a free man again... I mean free of worrying about the disease. Even though I thought he is free of cancer he was still thinking of how come the tumor is not gone!

He said there is a girl in Oregon with the same cancer and she is very brave too. She is surviving well without surgery and Chemo. She has the tumor too and it is not going away.

I was happy to know he is communicating with others about the cancer. So there were two people now we knew of who did not go for the chemo & surgery and the doctors way, and they were doing fine.

I continued travelling back and forth to Ecuador until Late 2017 When I moved back to California.

One day I noticed James's eating habit had Changed again, this time James was a raw eater, he looked even better with this new change.

He would take me along with him to some of the big hiking mountains in Palm Desert area, I loved the time I was spending with my son.

He was thinking California may not be the best place to live, so we took a few weeks and drove all the way to Dallas Texas and back, we saw so much, met many nice people.

Somehow we were so connected to California.

We came back to So. California and decided to stay put.

James said how about if you take care of Mia and I go travel and see what I need to do...I said Ok.

He decided to buy a RV and travel that way....Most

RVs had issues too. Too much plastic and glue... James was not going to take any unhealthy chances of anything.

So he just drove away with his regular car to places. He would come and visit every few weeks, that is what he is still doing. He comes and stays at the house for a week or two and then goes for a while.

I notice great changes when I see him...

Just a few months ago he stopped eating fruits too,...No watermelons anymore, no oranges ...not any kind of fruits ...Not even lemons...No Sugar at all...I did not know lemon has sugar!

He would not eat anything that would became sugar or had sugar in it.

He had finally found a way to get rid of the tumor!!! In a matter of just a few months, the tumor shrunk so much, now I do not even see the tumor any more, it seems this time it is gone!

James is following Hippocrates Institute method. He is growing sprouts, drinking his organic green juices and eating nuts & seeds. The nuts & seeds are organic, and raw and not pasteurized!!!! Very hard to find...Wow this is how he got rid of cancer!!!

He buys his produce from organic farmers directly.

His courage and discipline have provided him with this great life, free of cancer with total health.
I personally think he can eat things here and there, he says he does not want to change his taste buds.
James   in fact loves the vegetables and loves the smell of the herbs...How beautiful life is!!!!

I am so grateful for his recovery and it seems he has a better direction and a great future.

He is not working 8 to 5 and he is not struggling with traffic and he is not hustling like most young men are doing.

Money is not his focus, happiness is. With his degree in Chemical Engineering he could be making 6 figures
income but instead he is living very simple.   Beating cancer may be is "mastering life"!

He is a happy and content young man. He appreciates life. He is mindful and caring.

My friend Lesley smiling now and she is a changed person too. She says she is very grateful, she lives with gratitude and love, and compassion.

Side notes-

I learned you have to give it all to get rid of the disease!

Once one decides to live and makes the changes, the success will arrive fast!

I learned thinking good, seeing a good result in your mind makes days go by easier, chances are that is how everything changes for better.

Smiling and being supportive helps you and helps

the one who is healing.

Once you decide to make changes like: The food you put in your mouth, the soap you wash your body with, you are on your way to make your immune system good and strong to fight off the enemy cells.
Respecting your body is to support your body to fight back against unwated cells.
Instead of having chemicals attack all of the cells. To kill the bad and the good and may be by chance some good cells survive, and may be not, and then...
This is almost crazy and disrespectful to the body.

Drinking clean water, eating good food and staying away from all kinds of poison in the environment, will heal almost everything.

Most cancer patients die of other health issues and not
cancer itself, because the body gets treated by poisonous chemicals, the whole body gets damaged.
This action destroys other organs, when the organs get damaged by poison and medicine, anything can happen.
With chemicals the immune system gets destroyed and can not be helpful for survival. The damaged organs cause the death of the person, and not cancer

itself.

A friend was dignosed with cancer and went through all the regular treatments and within weeks the doctor said he is free of cancer. A few weeks later the cancer came back in another form and he got treated again. The doctor said again his body is free of cancer. In just a few more weeks the cancer came back but he died
before anymore treatments, his heart stopped working.

A teacher, hypnotherapy teacher in Napa, a city in northern California was diagnosed with cancer over 40 years ago. She said the doctor told her she will die in 2 or 3 months. Her daugether was 7 months pregnant then. She wanted to see her grand kid.
The doctor gave her an appointment for the next Monday to start the treatment so she could see her grand kid. The teacher was stunned, she said was num...She did not go to that apointment on that Monday or no other appointments after that...
She just decided not to do anything out of ordinary except she started eating better food. She sur-vivved and wrote a book about it! She is still living and
teaching.

There are so many crazy stories, the worst one is

when the doctor said to his patient, the worst thing you can do is to try to strengthen your immune system, that is a wrong thing to do! This is another crazy thing I have heard, not sure why a doctor would say this!

Everything written in this book, the whole content of this book is all true. The names are changed for privacy. This is what has happened to me for real, it can happen to anyone. I consider myself blessed to experience the results so good!
I hope this informtion to help people who are facing similar issues and need to decide. I hope they choose to respect their body and to take their time to do the right thing!

I have lost a few friends who gave into the system and they lost their lives. Some lasted a year or two and one lasted 3.5 years of harsh kind of living.
I have known people who have gone through the surgery but not the Chemo therapy and they have survived. One lived over 40 years after the surgery but had so many other health issues and struggled a lot and died at the age of 84.
Another lady I know who did the surgery over 40

years ago but changed many things and got away from bad food and bad water, she is still living and living well, better than most people her age.

Your thought determins your way of life, so think good thoughts no matter what.

Other notes-

I learned you do not get paid for family leave unless the person you are caring for, your loved one, goes through the system and gets regular treatments, by regular
doctors.
I had worked for 40+ years and paid taxes and all, and when I needed help the system was not available to me!

When you let others know about your challenge, real friends (the rare kind) stand by you and try to help.
Many friends (so called friends) stop calling you, many acquaintances stop calling you!
They just do not want to know! May be they think very
nagative about all of this!

Some friends & some relative do interfere & bad mouth you because to them this is crazy...I was criticized on

social media by my extended family member that if anything bad happens to James it will be my fault as if I forced James to go the natural way.

I did not encourage or discourage him because this is his life & he is a very intelligent man and he does not need my advice, I was just a support for him, to know he has me to lean on!

In business transactions, the ones who know about your ordeal may try to take advantage of you financially.

So. America, Ecuador Vilcabamba is beautiful, with great weather, great people, and cleaner air ...And very cheap .

The wifi works and everything else is also available and one can live there almost without worrying about money.